The Complete Carbohydrate Counter

Also in Pan Books

The Complete Calorie Counter
with an introduction by Eileen Fowler MBE

compiled by Kyle Cathie
with an introduction by
Katie Stewart

The complete
carbohydrate
counter

Pan Original Pan Books

First published 1978 by Pan Books

This revised edition published 1989 by Pan Books
an imprint of Pan Macmillan Ltd
Pan Macmillan, 20 New Wharf Road, London N1 9RR
Basingstoke and Oxford
Associated companies throughout the world
www.panmacmillan.com

ISBN 0 330 30726 6

16 18 17

A CIP catalogue record for this book is available from
the British Library.

Photoset by Parker Typesetting Service, Leicester
Printed and bound in Great Britain by
Mackays of Chatham PLC, Chatham, Kent

Contents

Introduction

It's hard to sort out just what you should and should not be eating, now that there seem to be so many conflicting theories about diet. But practical, good nutrition need not be dreary or difficult. It's simply a question of sticking to a steady pattern of balanced eating, one that includes a wide range of foods, to ensure that you get all the necessary nutrients for healthy living.

Carbohydrates are an essential part of the diet because they are a source of energy, but you have to watch them because carbohydrates eaten in excess of the body requirements are stored as fat. Carbohydrates (starches and sugars) are almost entirely the product of plants. Starches are found in cereals like wheat, rice, corn and oats, which means that foods based on these, such as pastry, cakes, bread, sauces thickened with flour, and rice dishes like risotto or kedgeree, and of course pasta dishes, are starchy foods. Starches are also found in root vegetables like potatoes, beetroot and turnips; beans, peas and other legumes are high in carbohydrates as well as protein. Most foods contain more than one nutrient but white sugar (sucrose) is pure carbohydrate and is used in the preparation of preserves, confectionery, suet puddings and desserts. You have to beware most of all of sugar, the consumption of which has increased enormously in Britain in the last century. Non-sugar sweeteners taste sweet, but bear no chemical or nutritional relationship to sugar and can be used when it's necessary to restrict the amount of carbohydrates in the diet. On the other hand it is better to cut out, or cut down on, these items altogether.

With this little book you can watch the amount of carbohydrates you are eating and, if necessary, reduce your carbohydrate intake. You will then be well on the way to having a trim figure. To keep a good shape you must know about the foods you eat, and a little of what you fancy will do you no harm at all.

The value of carbohydrate counting

There is only one way to lose weight and that is to eat less – a fundamental truth, you may say, but many of us find it difficult to do. Counting your carbohydrate intake is one of the easiest ways; not only are you counting in relatively low figures (whereas calories run into the thousands), but you are taking note of that part of any food you eat which, in the long run, actually turns into fat in the body. For anyone who's bad at sums, carbohydrate counting is a simple way of keeping a check on your weight or of dieting to lose extra kilogrammes.

Excess weight comes from taking in more energy in the food you eat than you use up in energy through both mental and physical exercise over a period. There should be an exact balance between the two for your weight to remain constant. Excess weight does not only come from eating too much food, but also from eating the wrong sorts of food – those with high carbohydrate and fat contents, rather than those with high protein values. To lose weight you have to break down the fat cells around the body by using up more energy in exercise than you absorb in food.

Foods are composed of three main constituents – carbohydrates, fats and proteins. The remainder is made up of small quantities of vitamins, amino acids, minerals and so on. There are very few foods which contain pure forms of carbohydrate, fat or protein. The carbohydrate content of a food is calculated by the amount of sugar, starch and dextrins that it contains. When digested, most of the carbohydrates are turned into glucose, which goes into the bloodstream. When we are eating a properly balanced diet, the glucose then forms our chief source of energy. But when the diet has too great a carbohydrate content the excess glucose goes to the liver where it is turned into fat and then stored around the body.

It is difficult to calculate the exact amount of energy we use up in physical and mental exercise during one day. A manual worker will obviously need more energy input than someone sitting at an office desk all day. An average 30-year-old man needs between 2,500 and 3,500 calories a day. A woman of the same age and of the right weight needs between 1,750 and 2,250 calories a day. A calorie is a unit of energy and one gramme of carbohydrate produces roughly four calories (one gramme of protein produces four calories, one gramme of fat nine).

Food containing 3,000 calories might be composed of 100 grammes of protein, 100 grammes of fat and 400 grammes of carbohydrate, so that a man's daily intake could be taken as 400 grammes of carbohydrate. For a woman eating food with a calorific value of, say, 2,000, the daily intake of carbohydrate could be taken as 250 grammes. These are average figures and you will have to work out for yourself whether your intake is higher or lower than the above figures. If you want to lose weight, try cutting your carbohydrate intake by 100 grammes a day over a period of two weeks. If you are not losing weight fast enough, try cutting your intake by a further 20 grammes. Trial and error will soon help you to work out a carbohydrate intake which suits your requirements.

The important thing to do is to set yourself a sensible target and then to stick to it for a couple of weeks, weighing yourself only three times during the period (at the beginning, after one week and after two weeks). Losing weight at the rate of 3·5 kilogrammes (8lb) a month is a manageable target to aim for.

It is of vital importance that you eat a well–balanced diet; by cutting out fats and carbohydrates completely you will not be eating a healthy diet and may well find yourself lacking in energy and constantly feeling tired and exhausted. There are two easily defined lists of foods which you can use when cutting down on carbohydrate intake:

Foods to eat in small quantities

bread of all kinds	potatoes
cereals	rice
cakes and biscuits	sugar
puddings	sweets and chocolates
pies and pastries	honey, jam and marmalade
pasta	alcohol and soft drinks

Foods to go for

meat	eggs
poultry and game	milk and cheese
fish	butter and margarine
vegetables	

Think carefully when you are preparing meals; could you substitute a second vegetable for potatoes at Sunday lunchtime? When eating out in a restaurant, could you ask for carrots or celery to nibble rather than eating a stodgy bread roll? Many of the snacks that we eat between meals – chocolates, nuts, crisps, biscuits and cakes – are high in carbohydrate content; be strong minded and try to avoid them completely.

There is much evidence to suggest that we eat more than is good for us. One good meal a day, taken either at lunchtime or in the evening, together with breakfast, tea and a light lunch or dinner depending on when you have your main meal, really is sufficient. You will be slightly more likely to lose weight if you take your main meal during the middle of the day, as you will have the remainder of the day to work off the carbohydrate intake in energy. There is little likelihood of the energy generated from a large meal in the evening being used up during your sleeping hours, although of course if you stayed in bed all day long you would still use up some energy.

Sugar is pure carbohydrate, and every effort should be made to cut down on the amount of sugar you eat if you are trying to lose weight. If you cannot do without it in tea or coffee, then try using sugar substitutes, which are available in both liquid and tablet form and which sweeten foods and contain no carbohydrates. Saccharin is a great boon to the slimmer. It can be used in powdered form on cereals, in liquid form on stewed fruits and in tablet form in drinks.

Weighing yourself daily when on a diet will not be encouraging. It is more effective to weigh yourself once a week and to keep a record of your progress to give encouragement. You will be at your lightest in the morning after you have been to the lavatory.

To sum up: if you want to lose weight, you need to expend more energy each day than you absorb. Cutting carbohydrates is one of the most successful methods of achieving this. Set yourself sensible targets, stick to them and you should be able to get down to your correct weight.

What you should weigh

Obviously this is only an approximate guide and is simply to give you some sort of target to work to. If you weigh yourself without clothes, then deduct about 1 kilogramme (2lb) from your weight as shown on the chart which follows. These weights are given for men and women over 25; deduct 0·5 kilogramme (1lb) for each year under 25 if you are between 18 and 24.

Women

Height		Small frame			Medium frame			Large frame		
ft in	cm	st	lb	kg	st	lb	kg	st	lb	kg
4 10	147·5	6	11	43	7	3	46	7	3	50·5
4 11	150	6	13	44	7	6	47	8	2	52
5 0	152·5	7	2	45·5	7	9	48·5	8	5	53
5 1	155	7	5	47	7	12	50	8	8	54·5
5 2	157·5	7	8	48	8	1	51	8	11	56
5 3	160	7	11	49·5	8	4	52·5	9	0	57
5 4	162·5	8	0	51	8	7	54	9	3	58·5
5 5	165	8	4	52·5	8	11	56	9	7	60
5 6	167.5	8	6	53·5	9	1	57·5	9	11	62
5 7	170	8	10	55	9	5	59·5	10	1	64
5 8	172·5	9	0	57	9	9	61	10	5	66
5 9	175	9	4	59	9	13	63	10	9	67·5
5 10	177·5	9	9	61	10	3	65	11	0	70
5 11	180	9	13	63	10	7	67	11	4	71·5
6 0	182·5	10	5	66	10	11	68·5	11	9	74

Men

Height		Small frame			Medium frame			Large frame		
ft in	cm	st	lb	kg	st	lb	kg	st	lb	kg
5 2	157·5	8	4	52·5	8	11	56	9	7	60
5 3	160	8	7	54	9	1	57·5	9	10	61·5
5 4	162·5	8	10	55	9	4	59	10	0	63·5
5 5	165	8	13	57	9	7	60	10	3	65
5 6	167·5	9	2	58	9	10	61·5	10	7	67
5 7	170	9	6	59·5	10	0	63·5	10	11	68·5
5 8	172·5	9	10	61·5	10	5	66	11	2	70·5
5 9	175	10	0	63·5	10	9	67·5	11	6	72·5
5 10	177·5	10	5	66	10	13	69	11	10	74
5 11	180	10	9	67·5	11	3	71	12	1	76·5
6 0	182·5	10	13	69	11	8	73	12	6	79
6 1	185	11	3	71	11	12	75	12	10	80·5
6 2	187·5	11	7	73	12	3	77·5	13	1	83
6 3	190	11	11	75	12	8	80	13	6	85
6 4	192·5	12	1	76·5	12	13	82	13	11	88

Carbohydrate counter

This chart gives the approximate carbohydrate content for 100 grammes and 1 ounce of the particular food. (Both figures have been given to the nearest whole number.)

Note Most carbohydrate values calculated for this book are taken from McCance and Widdowson's *The Composition of Foods*, fourth revised and extended edition of MRC Special Report No 297, by A. A. Paul and D. A. T. Southgate, issued by Her Majesty's Stationery Office.

	grammes of carbohydrate per 100g/per oz	
Aero	57	16
All–Bran	43	12
Almonds, fresh, shelled	4	1
Alpen	66	19
Angel Delight, per sachet, chocolate (made up)	16	5
Angel Delight, per sachet, raspberry (made up)	15	5
Apple, baked	10	3
Apple, cooking	10	3
Apple crumble	37	10
Apple, eating	12	4
Apple, dried	35	10
Apple dumpling	29	8
Apple juice	12	4
Apple pie	28	8
Apple pudding	30	8
Apple sauce	8	3
Apple, stewed, sweetened	17	5
Apple, stewed, unsweetened	8	3
Apricots, dried	43	12
Apricots, dried, stewed, unsweetened	16	5
Apricots, fresh	7	2
Apricots, stewed, sweetened	16	5
Apricots, stewed, unsweetened	6	2
Apricots, tinned in syrup	28	8
Apricots, tinned in fruit juice	8	3
Arrowroot, powder	94	27
Artichoke, globe, boiled	3	1
Artichoke, Jerusalem, boiled	3	1
Asparagus, boiled -	1	0·5

	grammes of carbohydrate per 100g/per oz	
Aubergine	3	1
Avocado pear, without dressing	2	1
Bacon	0	0
Baking powder	38	11
Banana, peeled	19	5
Banana custard	18	5
Barcelona nuts	5	2
Barley, creamed	95	27
Barley, pearl, raw	84	23
Barley, pearl, boiled	28	8
Barley water, lemon, concentrated	28	8
Bass	0	0
Beans, baked, tinned	10	3
Beans, broad, fresh, boiled	7	2
Beans, broad, raw	14	4
Beans, broad, tinned	7	2
Beans, butter, raw	50	14
Beans, butter, fresh, boiled	17	5
Beans, butter, tinned	16	5
Beans, French, boiled	1	0·5
Beans, green, runner, boiled	3	1
Beans, green, runner, frozen, boiled	4	1
Beans, green, runner, tinned	1	0·5
Beans, haricot, boiled	17	5
Beans, red kidney	45	13
Beans and burgers, tinned	9	3
Beans and sausages, tinned	14	4
Beansprouts	1	0·5
Beef, generally	0	0
Beef, braised slices, frozen	2	1

	grammes of carbohydrate per 100g/per oz	
Beef, corned, without sugar	0	0
Beef sausages, fried or grilled	15	5
Beef stew	4	1
Beefburgers, fried or grilled	7	2
Beefsteak pie	21	6
Beefsteak pudding	19	5
Beetroot, boiled	10	3
Bemax	45	13
Bilberries, raw	14	4
Biscuits, Cheddars	55	16
Biscuits, cream crackers	68	19
Biscuits, digestive	66	19
Biscuits, digestive, chocolate	67	19
Biscuits, fig roll	69	20
Biscuits, Garibaldi	69	20
Biscuits, ginger snaps	79	23
Biscuits, Hobnobs	71	20
Biscuits, petit beurre	78	22
Biscuits, plain	70	20
Biscuits, sponge fingers	79	23
Biscuits, sweet	62	18
Biscuits, Tuc Sandwich	54	15
Biscuits, vanilla wafers	66	19
Biscuits, water	76	21
Blackberries, fresh, unsweetened	6	2
Blackberries, stewed, sweetened	15	5
Blackberries, stewed, unsweetened	5	2
Blackberries, tinned in fruit juice	9	3
Blackcurrants, puréed	40	11
Blackcurrants, raw, unsweetened	6	2
Blackcurrants, stewed, sweetened	15	5

grammes of carbohydrate	per 100g	per oz
Blackcurrants, stewed, unsweetened	7	2
Blackcurrant tarts	57	16
Blackcurrants, tinned	25	7
Black pudding, fried	15	5
Blancmange, made up	19	5
Bloater, grilled	0	0
Boiled sweets	87	25
Bolognese sauce	2	1
Bounty bar	58	17
Bournvita	79	23
Bovril meat extract	3	1
Brains	0	0
Bran, wheat	27	8
Brawn	0	0
Brazil nuts, shelled	2	1
Bread, brown	50	14
Bread, currant	52	15
Bread, fried, white	51	15
Bread, Hovis	68	19
Bread, malt	49	14
Bread sauce	13	4
Bread, soda	56	16
Bread, starch-reduced rolls	46	13
Bread, toasted, white	65	18
Bread, white	50	14
Bread, wholemeal	42	12
Bread and butter pudding	17	5
Breadcrumbs, dried	77	22
Bream	0	0
Brill	0	0
Broccoli, fresh, boiled	2	1

grammes of carbohydrate	per 100g	per oz
Broccoli, packet, frozen	4	1
Brown sauce, bottled	25	7
Brussels sprouts, fresh, boiled	2	1
Brussels sprouts, frozen	11	3
Buck rarebit	17	5
Buckwheat, raw	70	20
Buckwheat, cooked	25	7
Buns, Bath	60	17
Buns, currant	54	15
Butter	trace	trace
Butter, peanut, smooth	13	4
Buttermilk	4	1
Cabbage, red, raw	4	1
Cabbage, red, pickled	trace	trace
Cabbage, Savoy, boiled	1	0·5
Cabbage, Savoy, raw	3	1
Cambridge loaf	28	8
Canary pudding	56	16
Carrots, new, tinned	4	1
Carrots, old, boiled	4	2
Carrots, old, raw	5	2
Cashew nuts, salted	25	7
Castle pudding	47	13
Catfish, fried	6	2
Catfish, steamed or grilled	0	0
Cauliflower, fresh, boiled	1	0·5
Cauliflower, fresh, raw	2	1
Cauliflower cheese	5	2
Celeriac, boiled	2	1
Celery, boiled or braised	1	0·5

grammes of carbohydrate	per 100g	per oz
Celery, raw	1	0·5
Chapatis, made with fat	50	14
Chapatis, made without fat	44	12
Cheese, generally	trace	trace
Cheese, cottage	7	2
Cheese, Norwegian Mysost	43	12
Cheese omelette	trace	trace
Cheese pudding	8	3
Cheese sauce	9	3
Cheese spread	1	0·5
Cheese straws	26	7
Cheeseburgers	60	17
Cheesecake	24	7
Cherries, fresh, raw	12	4
Cherries, fresh, stewed, sweetened	20	6
Cherries, fresh, stewed, unsweetened	10	3
Cherries, glacé	56	16
Cherry and coconut cake	57	16
Chestnuts, shelled	37	10
Chicken, generally	0	0
Chicken casserole	21	6
Chicken curry	8	3
Chicken pie	27	8
Chicken rissoles	21	6
Chicken soup, tinned	5	2
Chicken spread	11	3
Chicken supreme, tinned	4	1
Chicken and ham pie	22	6
Chicken and mushroom casserole	4	1
Chicken and noodle soup mix, made up	4	1
Chicory, raw	2	1

grammes of carbohydrate	per 100g	per oz
Chives	0	0
Chocolate biscuits	67	19
Chocolate cup cakes	77	22
Chocolate, drinking, powder	74	21
Chocolate, fancy	73	21
Chocolate, fruit and nut	51	15
Chocolate, milk	59	17
Chocolate mousse (Chambourcy)	29	8
Chocolate, plain	65	18
Chocolate pudding	44	12
Chocolate spread	70	20
Chocolate, whole nut	48	14
Chop suey	21	6
Chow mein	14	4
Christmas pudding	48	14
Chutney, apple	50	14
Chutney, sweet mango	60	17
Chutney, tomato	40	11
Cob nuts, shelled	7	2
Coca-cola	10	3
Cockles	trace	trace
Cocoa, powder	11	3
Coconut cake	53	15
Coconut cream	70	20
Coconut, desiccated	6	2
Coconut, fresh	4	1
Coconut milk	5	1
Cod, baked	0	0
Cod, fillets, frozen	0	0
Cod, fried in batter	7	2
Cod, grilled	0	0

	grammes of carbohydrate per 100g/per oz	
Cod, roe, baked in vinegar	0	0
Cod, roe, fried	3	1
Cod liver oil	0	0
Coffee, black, made up	trace	trace
Coffee and chicory essence	56	16
Coleslaw	9	3
Complan (Glaxo)	35	13
Conger eel, steamed or grilled	0	0
Conger eel, fried	7	2
Cooking fat	0	0
Corn oil	0	0
Corn on the cob	23	7
Corned beef (Fray Bentos)	0	0
Cornflakes	85	24
Cornflour	92	25
Cornish pasties	31	9
Cottage pie	9	3
Courgettes	0	0
Crab, boiled	0	0
Cranberries, fresh	4	1
Cranberry sauce	46	13
Cream, fresh, double	2	1
Cream, fresh, single	3	1
Cream, fresh, whipping	3	1
Cream, whipping, longlife	3	1
Cream, soured	2	1
Cream, tinned, single	3	1
Cream, top of the milk	3	1
Cream, imitation	8	3
Cress	trace	trace
Crispbread, wheat, starch-reduced	37	10

grammes of carbohydrate	per 100g	per oz
Crispbread, rye	71	20
Crisps, potato	49	14
Crumpets	37	10
Crunchie bar (per bar)	31	9
Cucumber, raw	2	1
Currant buns	54	15
Currant cake	64	18
Currants, dried	63	18
Curried meat	8	3
Curry powder	26	7
Custard, apple	18	5
Custard, baked egg	11	3
Custard powder, made up	17	5
Custard powder, raw	92	26
Custard pudding, baked	35	10
Custard tart	30	9
Dabs, fried	8	3
Damsons, fresh, raw	10	3
Damsons, fresh, stewed, sweetened	18	5
Damsons, fresh, stewed, unsweetened	8	3
Damsons, tinned	7	2
Dates, fresh, weighed with stones	55	16
Dates, dried, stoned	64	18
Dogfish, fried	7	2
Dogfish, steamed or grilled	0	0
Doughnuts	49	14
Dripping, beef	0	0
Duck	0	0
Dumplings	25	7
Dundee cake	62	18

	grammes of carbohydrate per 100g/per oz	
Easter biscuit	68	19
Eccles cakes	51	15
Eclairs	38	11
Eels	0	0
Eggs, boiled, fried, poached or scrambled	trace	trace
Egg sauce	9	2
Egg, Scotch	12	3
Endive	1	0·5
Energen rolls	46	13
Faggots	15	5
Farex	76	22
Figs, dried, raw	53	15
Figs, dried, stewed, sweetened	34	9
Figs, dried, stewed, unsweetened	29	8
Figs, fresh	10	3
Fish cakes, fried	15	5
Fish fingers, fried	17	5
Fish paste	4	1
Flake (per bar)	20	6
Flounder, fried	7	2
Flounder, steamed or grilled	0	0
Flour, wholemeal (100%)	66	19
Flour, brown (85%)	69	20
Flour, white (72%), breadmaking	75	21
Flour, household, plain	80	23
Flour, self-raising	77	22
Flour, patent (40%)	78	22
Frankfurter	3	1
French dressing	0	0
Fruit cake, rich	58	17

grammes of carbohydrate	per 100g	per oz
Fruit cake, rich, iced	62	18
Fruit gums	63	18
Fruit mousses	25	7
Fruit pie, individual, pastry	57	16
Fruit salad, tinned in syrup	25	7
Fruit salad, tinned in juice	10	3
Fruit squash, undiluted	28	8
Fruit squash, diluted	11	3
Fudge	99	28
Gammon	0	0
Genoa cake	53	15
Gherkins	trace	trace
Ginger biscuits	79	23
Ginger, ground	60	17
Gingerbread	63	18
Glucose	85	24
Goose	0	0
Gooseberries, fresh	3	1
Gooseberries, stewed, sweetened	12	4
Gooseberries, stewed, unsweetened	3	1
Gooseberries, tarts	57	16
Gooseberries, tinned	18	5
Gooseberry pie	28	8
Grape juice, red	16	5
Grape juice, white	15	5
Grapefruit, fresh, unsweetened	3	1
Grapefruit juice, tinned, sweetened	10	3
Grapefruit juice, tinned, unsweetened	8	3
Grapefruit squash, concentrated	36	10
Grapefruit squash, diluted	25	7

grammes of carbohydrate per 100g/per oz		
Grapefruit, tinned	15	5
Grapenuts	76	22
Grapes, black, fresh	13	4
Grapes, green, fresh	15	5
Greengages, fresh, unstoned	11	3
Greengages, stewed, sweetened	19	5
Greengages, stewed, unsweetened	7	2
Grouse	0	0
Guinea fowl	0	0
Gurnet, red or grey	0	0
Haddock, fried	4	1
Haddock, fried and breadcrumbed	11	3
Haddock, smoked	0	0
Haddock, steamed	0	0
Haggis	19	5
Hake, fried	5	1
Hake, fried and breadcrumbed	7	2
Hake, steamed	0	0
Halibut	0	0
Ham	0	0
Ham and beef roll	14	4
Ham and pork, chopped loaf	0	0
Hamburger	4	1
Hare	0	0
Hazel nuts, shelled	7	2
Heart, pig's, ox or sheep's	0	0
Herring, baked or grilled	0	0
Herring, fried	1	0·5
Herring roe, fried	5	1
Honey	76	22

	grammes of carbohydrate per 100g/per oz	
Honeycomb	74	21
Horlicks	73	21
Horseradish, raw	11	3
Horseradish sauce	25	7
Hot-pot, Lancashire	10	3
Ice-cream, dairy	25	7
Ice-cream, non-dairy	21	6
Icing	88	25
Instant Whip, fruit, made up	95	27
Irish stew	7	2
Jaffa juice, orange squash, tinned	11	3
Jam, generally	69	20
Jam, reduced sugar	33	9
Jam, omelette	27	8
Jam roll (Swiss)	63	18
Jam tarts	63	18
Jelly, raw, fruit	63	18
Jelly, made up	14	4
Jelly, milk	16	5
John Dory	0	0
Junket	14	4
Kedgeree	9	3
Ketchup, tomato	24	7
Kidneys	0	0
Kippers	0	0
KitKat (per bar)	31	9
Kohlrabi	4	1

	grammes of carbohydrate per 100g/per oz	
Lamb	0	0
Lard	0	0
Laverbread	2	1
Leeks, boiled	5	1
Leeks, raw	6	2
Lemon, fresh	3	1
Lemon barley water, concentrated	28	8
Lemon curd, homemade	41	12
Lemon curd, starch based	63	18
Lemon curd tarts	50	14
Lemon juice, fresh	2	1
Lemon meringue pie	46	13
Lemon sole, steamed or grilled	0	0
Lemon sole, fried	9	3
Lemonade, bought	6	2
Lemonade, homemade	13	4
Lemonade shandy	18	5
Lemon squash, concentrated	21	6
Lentils, boiled	17	5
Lentils, dried, uncooked	53	15
Lentil soup	12	4
Lettuce	1	0·5
Limes	4	1
Lime juice cordial, undiluted	30	9
Ling, steamed or grilled	0	0
Ling, fried	6	2
Lion Bar (per bar)	33	9
Liquorice all-sorts	74	21
Liver, calf, fried	7	2
Liver, chicken, fried	3	1
Liver, lamb, fried	4	1

grammes of carbohydrate per 100g/per oz		
Liver, ox, stewed	4	1
Liver, pig's, stewed	4	1
Liver sausage	4	1
Lobster, boiled	trace	trace
Loganberries, raw	3	1
Loganberries, stewed, sweetened	13	4
Loganberries, stewed, unsweetened	3	1
Loganberries, tinned in syrup	26	7
Low-fat spread	0	0
Lucozade	18	5
Luncheon meat	5	2
Luncheon meat, roll	25	7
Lychees, fresh	16	5
Lychees, tinned	18	5
Macaroni, boiled	25	7
Macaroni cheese	15	4
Macaroni cheese, tinned	11	3
Macaroni, creamed	14	4
Macaroni, raw	79	22
Mackerel	0	0
Madeira cake	58	17
Malted milk	70	20
Maltesers	61	17
Mandarins, tinned	14	4
Mango, fresh	15	5
Mango, tinned	20	6
Margarine (all kinds)	0	0
Marmalade	70	20
Marmalade, reduced sugar	33	9
Marmite	2	1

grammes of carbohydrate per	100g	per oz
Marrow, boiled	1	0·5
Mars bar	66	19
Marshmallows	85	24
Marvel, milk powder	53	15
Marzipan	49	14
Mayonnaise	0	0
Meat balls, in gravy	6	2
Meat paste	3	1
Medlars	11	3
Melon, cantaloup	3	1
Melon, honeydew	3	1
Melon, watermelon	3	1
Meringues	96	27
Milk, fresh, dairy	5	1
Milk, condensed, full cream, sweetened	55	16
Milk, condensed, skimmed, sweetened	60	17
Milk, evaporated, unsweetened	11	3
Milk, instant	53	15
Milk powder, full cream	39	11
Milk powder, low fat	53	15
Milk, skimmed	5	1
Mincemeat	62	18
Mince pies	62	18
Minestrone, dried mix, made up	4	1
Minstrels	67	19
Mint, fresh	39	11
Mint sauce	35	10
Mints, After Eight Thin	76	22
Mints, glacier (Fox's)	99	28
Mixed fruit pudding	46	13
Mixed peel, candied	66	19

grammes of carbohydrate per	100g	per oz
Molasses	67	19
Monkfish, fried	5	2
Monkfish, steamed or grilled	0	0
Moussaka	10	3
Muesli	66	19
Mulberries	8	2
Mullet, red or grey	0	0
Mushrooms, raw or fried	0	0
Mushroom soup, tinned	4	1
Mussels	trace	trace
Mustard and cress, raw	1	0.5
Mustard powder	21	6
Mutton, generally	0	0
Mutton chop, fried	6	2
Nectarines	11	3
Nescafé, black, made up	trace	trace
Nescafé, powder	11	3
Noodles, cooked	28	8
Noodles, raw	81	23
Nutmeat, Granose	11	3
Nutmeat, brawn	5	2
Oatcakes	63	18
Oatmeal porridge, boiled	8	2
Oil, cooking, olive and vegetable	0	0
Okra	2	1
Olives, black and green	trace	trace
Omelette, plain	trace	trace
Onion, boiled	3	1
Onion, fried	10	3

	grammes of carbohydrate per 100g/per oz	
Onion, pickled	4	1
Onion, raw	5	2
Onion sauce	8	3
Onion, spring	8	2
Opal fruits	91	26
Orange, fresh, whole	6	2
Orange cake, iced	63	18
Orange juice, fresh	9	3
Orange juice, tinned, unsweetened	8	3
Orange squash, concentrated	36	10
Orange squash, tinned	11	3
Outline low-calorie fat spread	0	0
Ovaltine, powder	81	23
Oxo cubes	12	4
Oxtail	0	0
Oxtail soup, tinned	5	2
Ox tongue	0	0
Oysters, raw	trace	trace
Paella	14	4
Pancakes	36	10
Parsley, fresh	trace	trace
Parsnip, boiled	14	4
Parsnip, raw	11	3
Partridge	0	0
Passion fruit	3	1
Pasta, lasagne, uncooked	70	20
Pasta, quill, cooked	32	9
Pasta, quill, uncooked	77	22
Pasta, rigatoni, uncooked	70	20
Pasta, shells, cooked	34	9

grammes of carbohydrate	per 100g	per oz
Pasta, shells, uncooked	77	22
Pasta, spaghetti, cooked	23	7
Pasta, wholewheat instant spirals, uncooked	52	15
Pastilles	62	18
Pastry, choux, baked	31	9
Pastry, flaky, baked	47	13
Pastry, shortcrust, baked	56	16
Pâté	11	3
Pawpaw, tinned	17	5
Peach, fresh	9	3
Peach, dried	53	15
Peach, dried, stewed, unsweetened	20	6
Peach, stewed, sweetened	23	7
Peach, tinned in syrup	23	7
Peach, tinned in fruit juice	9	3
Peanut butter, smooth	13	4
Peanut butter, crunchy	13	4
Peanuts, shelled, salted	9	3
Pear, fresh	11	3
Pear, dried, stewed, unsweetened	18	5
Pear, stewed, sweetened	17	5
Pear, stewed, unsweetened	8	3
Pear, tinned in syrup	20	6
Pear, tinned in fruit juice	9	3
Peas, dried, boiled	19	5
Peas, fresh, raw	11	3
Peas, fresh, boiled	8	2
Peas, frozen, boiled	4	1
Pea soup, thick	52	15
Peas, split, boiled	22	6

	grammes of carbohydrate per 100g/per oz	
Peas, tinned, garden	7	2
Peas, tinned, processed	14	4
Pease pudding	15	5
Pepper, black or white	68	20
Peppers, red or green, raw	2	1
Peppermints	102	29
Pheasant	0	0
Pickle, mustard (Heinz)	26	7
Pickle, piccalilli	6	2
Pickle, ploughman's (Heinz)	31	10
Pickle, sweet	34	9
Pickle, tomato (Heinz)	24	7
Pickled onions	4	1
Pickled walnuts	7	2
Pigeon	0	0
Pilchard	0	0
Pineapple, fresh, weighed with skin	11	3
Pineapple juice, tinned	13	4
Pineapple squash	18	5
Pineapple, tinned in syrup	20	6
Pineapple, tinned in juice	16	5
Pizza (Bird's Eye)	25	7
Plaice, steamed or grilled	0	0
Plaice, fried in batter	14	4
Plaice, fried and breadcrumbed	9	3
Plantain, boiled	31	9
Plantain, fried	47	13
PLJ	4	1
Plums, fresh, dessert, unstoned	9	3
Plums, cooking, stewed, sweetened	15	5
Plums, cooking, stewed, unsweetened	5	2

grammes of carbohydrate per 100g/per oz		
Plums, pie	28	8
Plums, red, tinned	17	5
Plum pudding	53	15
Pollack, steamed or grilled	0	0
Polony	14	4
Pontefract cake	70	20
Pork, generally	0	0
Pork pie	25	7
Porridge, made up	8	2
Porridge instant oats	70	20
Potato, baked	25	7
Potato, boiled, new	18	5
Potato, boiled, old	20	6
Potato, chipped, frozen	29	8
Potato, chipped, old	37	11
Potato crisps	49	14
Potato, instant, made up	16	5
Potato, mashed	18	5
Potato, roast, old	27	8
Potato soup	11	3
Potato, tinned, new	13	4
Prawns	0	0
Prunes, dried, unstoned	34	9
Prunes, dried, stewed, unsweetened	20	5
Prunes, tinned in juice	31	9
Prunes, tinned in syrup	25	7
Puffed Wheat	68	19
Pumpkin	3	1
Quaker Oats, raw	67	19
Queen cakes	58	17

	grammes of carbohydrate per 100g/per oz	
Queen of Puddings	34	9
Quiche Lorraine	21	6
Quince, fresh	6	2
Rabbit	0	0
Radish, raw	3	1
Raisins, dried	64	18
Raisins, dried, seedless	70	20
Raspberries, fresh	6	2
Raspberries, frozen	7	2
Raspberries, stewed, sweetened	17	5
Raspberries, stewed, unsweetened	6	2
Raspberries, tinned in syrup	22	6
Ravioli, tinned	14	4
Ready Brek	70	20
Red currants	4	1
Revels	64	18
Rhubarb, fresh, stewed, sweetened	11	3
Rhubarb, fresh, stewed, unsweetened	1	0·5
Rhubarb pie	28	8
Rhubarb, tinned in syrup	7	2
Ribena, concentrated	61	17
Ribena, diluted	21	6
Rice, boiled	30	8
Rice, creamed	16	5
Rice, ground	81	23
Rice pudding, tinned	15	5
Rice, raw	87	25
Rice Krispies	88	25
Rissoles, fried	21	6
Rock cakes	60	17

grammes of carbohydrate	per 100g	per oz
Roe, cod's, fried	3	1
Rosehip syrup, concentrated	62	18
Rye flour (100%)	76	22
Ryvita	66	19
Sago, raw	94	27
Sago, creamed	11	3
Sago, creamed, tinned	11	3
Sago pudding	20	6
Saithe	0	0
Salad cream	15	5
Salad dressing	0	0
Salami	2	1
Salmon	0	0
Salsify, boiled	3	1
Salt	0	0
Sardines	0	0
Sausages, pork, fried or grilled	11	3
Sausages, beef, fried or grilled	15	5
Sausages, black	15	4
Sausages, liver	4	1
Sausages, luncheon meat	5	2
Sausage rolls	36	10
Saveloy	10	3
Scallops	trace	trace
Scampi, boiled	0	0
Scampi, fried	29	8
Scones	56	16
Scotch broth, tinned	6	2
Scotch egg	12	4
Scotch pancakes	41	11

	grammes of carbohydrate per 100g/per oz	
Seakale, boiled	1	0·5
Semolina, raw	78	22
Semolina, creamed	11	3
Semolina pudding	20	6
Shepherd's pie	9	3
Shortbread	65	18
Shredded Wheat	68	19
Shreddies	73	21
Shrimps	0	0
Skate, fried	4	1
Skate, grilled or steamed	0	0
Smarties (per tube)	28	8
Smelts, fried	4	1
Sole, lemon, fried	9	3
Sole, lemon, grilled or steamed	0	0
Soya flour, full fat	23	7
Soya flour, low fat	28	8
Spaghetti, raw	84	24
Spaghetti, cooked, plain	26	7
Spaghetti Bolognese, tinned	13	4
Spaghetti, tinned, with tomato sauce	12	4
Special K	78	22
Spinach, fresh, boiled	1	0·5
Spinach, frozen	14	4
Sponge cake, made with fat	53	15
Sponge cake, made without fat	54	15
Sponge cake, with jam	64	18
Sponge pudding, steamed	46	13
Sprats	0	0
Spring greens, boiled	1	0·5
Spry cooking fat	0	0

	grammes of carbohydrate per 100g/per oz	
Steak	0	0
Steak, stewed with gravy	1	0·5
Steak and kidney pie	16	5
Stock cubes	12	4
Strawberries, fresh	6	2
Strawberries, frozen	11	3
Strawberries, tinned in syrup	21	6
Stuffing, country	80	23
Sturgeon	trace	trace
Suet	0	0
Suet, shredded	12	4
Suet pudding	41	11
Sugar, all kinds	105	30
Sugar Puffs	84	24
Sultanas	65	18
Swedes, boiled	4	1
Sweetbreads, fried	6	2
Sweetcorn, on-the-cob, boiled	23	7
Sweetcorn, tinned	16	5
Sweet potatoes, boiled	20	6
Syrup, golden	79	22
Syrup, golden, pudding	79	23
Tangerines, fresh, weighed with skins	6	2
Tapioca, raw	95	27
Tapioca, creamed	14	4
Tapioca pudding	21	6
Tea, without milk	trace	trace
Toad-in-the-hole	19	6
Toast, white	65	18
Toffee	71	26

	grammes of carbohydrate per 100g/per oz	
Toffee Crisp (per bar)	30	9
Tomato, fresh, raw	3	1
Tomato, fresh, fried	3	1
Tomato juice, tinned	3	1
Tomato ketchup	24	7
Tomato purée	11	3
Tomato sauce	8	3
Tomato soup, tinned	6	3
Tomatoes, tinned	2	1
Tongue, boiled	0	0
Tongue, ox	0	0
Topic (per bar)	27	8
Treacle, black	67	19
Treacle pudding	51	15
Treacle tart	61	17
Trifle	24	7
Tripe	0	0
Trout	0	0
Tuna, fresh or tinned	0	0
Turbot, steamed	0	0
Turbot, grilled or fried	6	2
Turkey	0	0
Turkish delight (Fry's), per bar	38	11
Turnips, boiled	2	1
Turnip tops, boiled	trace	trace
Veal, fried	4	1
Veal, stewed	0	0
Vegetable soup, tinned	7	2
Vegetable spaghetti	4	1
Vegetable oil	0	0

	grammes of carbohydrate per 100g/per oz	
Venison	0	0
Vermicelli, raw	81	23
Vermicelli, cooked	28	8
Victoria sandwich	64	18
Vinegar	1	0·5
Virol	60	17
Vita-Weat	78	22
Walnuts, shelled	5	1
Watercress, fresh	1	0·5
Weetabix	70	20
Welsh cheesecakes	60	17
Welsh rarebit	24	7
Wheat germ	53	15
Whelks	trace	trace
Whitebait, fried	5	2
Whitebait, steamed or boiled	0	0
Whiting, fried	7	2
Whiting, steamed or boiled	0	0
White sauce, savoury	11	3
White sauce, sweet	19	5
Winkles	trace	trace
Wispa (per bar)	19	5
Witch, fried	7	2
Witch, steamed or boiled	0	0
Yams, boiled	30	9
Yeast, baker's	1	0·5
Yeast, dried	3	1
Yoghurt, natural	6	2
Yoghurt, flavoured	14	4

	grammes of carbohydrate per 100g/per oz	
Yoghurt, fruit	18	5
Yoghurt, hazelnut	16	5
Yorkshire pudding	26	7

Alcoholic drinks

All measurements are either standard can sizes or standard pub measurements.

Beer	measure	grammes of carbohydrate
Brown ale	1 pint	40
Draught bitter	1 pint	42
Draught mild	1 pint	35
Guinness, draught and bottled	1 pint	17
Lager	1 pint	38
Pale ale	1 pint	45
Shandy	11·5 fl oz	28
Stout	1 pint	53
Strong	⅓ pint	33

Cider		
Dry	1 pint	53
Sweet	1 pint	63
Vintage	1 pint	70

Spirits		
Bourbon	⅙ gill	15
Brandy	⅙ gill	20
Campari	⅓ gill	30
Gin	⅙ gill	13
Vermouth, dry	⅓ gill	15
Vermouth, sweet	⅓ gill	20
Vodka	⅙ gill	15
Whisky	⅙ gill	15

Wines	measure	grammes of carbohydrate
Dry	4 fl oz	25
Sweet	4 fl oz	28
Champagne	4 fl oz	20
Port	⅓ gill	20
Sherry, dry	⅓ gill	15
Sherry, sweet	⅓ gill	15

Soft drinks		
Bitter lemon	11·5 fl oz	28
Coca-cola	11·5 fl oz	33
Dry ginger	11·5 fl oz	13
Ginger beer	9·6 fl oz	30
Grapefruit juice	4 fl oz	12
Lemon juice	4 fl oz	3
Lemonade	1 pint	33
Lucozade	4 fl oz	20
Orange juice	4 fl oz	15
Tomato juice	4 fl oz	5
Tonic water	11·5 fl oz	23

Recipes

Soups and starters

Artichoke soup

Serves 4   carbohydrates per portion: 15

450 g (1 lb) Jerusalem artichokes
1 large onion
50 g (2 oz) butter
600 ml (1 pint) chicken stock
150 ml (¼ pint) milk
salt, pepper and a pinch of nutmeg

Wash the artichokes and make sure that you get rid of all the dirt; there is no need to peel them. Slice them roughly. Peel and finely slice the onion. Melt the butter in a large saucepan and add the onion. Leave to soften and then add the artichokes. Stir thoroughly so that they become coated with the butter. Add the stock, salt, pepper and nutmeg and bring to the boil. Simmer for about 15–20 minutes until the artichokes are soft. Put the soup through a mouli or blender. Return to the pan, stir in the milk and adjust the seasoning. Serve hot.

Watercress soup

Serves 4   carbohydrates per portion: 8

2 bunches watercress
25 g (1 oz) butter
1 medium-sized potato

600 ml (1 pint) chicken stock
150 ml (¼ pint) milk
Salt and pepper

Wash the watercress and keep two or three stalks for garnishing. Take out any tough-looking stalks and chop the watercress roughly. Melt the butter in a large saucepan and add the watercress. Stir and leave for five minutes. Scrub the potato and dice finely. Add to the pan, stir and then pour in the stock. Season with salt and pepper. Bring to the boil, simmer for 30 minutes or until the potato is cooked and put through a mouli or blender. Return to the pan, stir in the milk and adjust the seasoning if necessary. Pour into hot bowls and garnish with watercress leaves.

Tomato soup

Serves 4   carbohydrates per portion: 17

675 g (1½ lb) tomatoes
1 large onion
50 g (2 oz) lean bacon
2 tablespoons olive oil
1 teaspoon sugar
1 large potato
600 ml (1 pint) chicken stock
1 tablespoon chives, finely chopped
2 tablespoons sour cream
salt and pepper

Stand the tomatoes in boiling water for 30 seconds, pierce the skins, drain and peel. Chop roughly. Peel and finely slice the onion. Roughly chop the bacon. Heat the olive oil in a large saucepan and add the onion and bacon. Allow to soften but not burn. Add the tomatoes and sprinkle with the sugar. Add the potato, scrubbed thoroughly and diced finely, and leave to cook for 5 minutes. Then pour over the stock, season with salt and pepper, and bring to the boil. Leave to simmer for 30 minutes or until the potato and tomatoes are soft. Put the soup through a mouli or blender. Pour back into the pan, adjust seasoning and pour into hot bowls. Garnish each with half a tablespoon of sour cream and a sprinkling of chives.

Marinated kipper fillets

Serves 4   carbohydrates per portion: 4

1 packet boned kipper fillets
1 small onion
1 bay leaf
1 teaspoon sugar

4 tablespoons olive oil
3 tablespoons wine vinegar
salt and pepper

Using a sharp knife, strip the skin from each kipper fillet. Cut the fish into 4-cm (1½-in) lengths. Cut the onion into rings and arrange in a dish with the fish. Put the bay leaf in the middle. Mix the remaining ingredients together and pour over the kippers. Leave in a cool place for at least three or four hours before serving with slices of brown bread and butter.

Main courses

Haricot beans with anchovies

Serves 4   carbohydrates per portion: 25

450 g (1 lb) haricot beans, soaked in water overnight
3 medium-sized onions
3 tablespoons olive oil
6 anchovies, chopped roughly
150 ml (¼ pint) liquor in which beans are cooked
the juice of 1 lemon
1 tablespoon finely chopped parsley
salt, pepper and freshly grated nutmeg

Drain the beans, refill the pot with cold water and bring to the boil. Simmer for about 1½ hours or until tender. Salt should be added about half-way through the cooking time. When the beans are almost cooked, finely slice the onions and fry them gently in the olive oil. Add the remaining ingredients and allow to heat through thoroughly. Mix with the beans and serve, the hotter the better.

Cheese, egg and bean salad

Serves 4   carbohydrates per portion: 5

4 eggs
4 lettuce leaves
450 g (1 lb) French beans
450 g (1 lb) cottage cheese
1 large or 2 small red peppers

Hard boil the eggs, shell them and cut into quarters. Arrange the lettuce leaves on the plates. Boil the French beans in lightly salted water for 10 minutes or until tender. Drain them and arrange around the edge of the lettuce leaves. Mound the cottage cheese in the middle of each leaf, and decorate with the quartered eggs and the red peppers, which should be deseeded and cut into fine strips.

Cauliflower cheese

Serves 4   carbohydrates per portion: 17

1 cauliflower, weighing about 675 g (1½ lb)
1 egg
600 ml (1 pint) low-fat milk
25 g (1 oz) butter
100 g (4 oz) strong English Cheddar, grated
salt and pepper

Wash the cauliflower and cut off the outer leaves. Plunge it into lightly salted, boiling water and cook for about 15–20 minutes or until tender but not breaking up. Drain. While the cauliflower is cooking, make the cheese sauce as follows: put the egg, milk and butter in a bowl over a saucepan of hot, but not boiling, water. Stir continuously until you have a smooth sauce. Add three-quarters of the cheese and season with salt and pepper. Pour this sauce over the cooked cauliflower, which should have been placed in an ovenproof dish, and sprinkle with the remaining cheese. Bake in a hot oven (200°C, 400°F, Gas 6) for ten minutes, or brown under a hot grill.

Goulash

Serves 3   carbohydrates per portion: 20

50 g (2 oz) fat bacon
1 large onion, finely sliced
1 clove garlic, peeled and chopped
450 g (1 lb) beef, topside or stewing steak
1 tablespoon flour
1 glass red wine
150 ml (¼ pint) stock
1 bouquet garni
salt, pepper and paprika pepper

Chop the bacon roughly. Heat a little fat in a medium-sized saucepan and add the bacon, onion and garlic. Fry gently for 5 minutes until softened but not browned. Add the beef, which should have been cut into cubes and sprinkled with flour. Stir vigorously until browned all over. Pour over the red wine and the stock. Add the bouquet garni and season liberally with paprika pepper and salt and pepper. Put into the oven (150°C, 300°F, Gas 2) or simmer gently on top of the stove for 1–1½ hours. Remove the bouquet garni and serve.

Toad-in-the-hole

Serves 2   carbohydrates per portion: 25

300 ml (½ pint) milk   25 g (1 oz) dripping
100 g (4 oz) flour   225 g (8 oz) pork sausages
2 eggs   salt and pepper

Make a batter mixture from the milk, flour and eggs. Season with salt and pepper and pour into a small tin containing hot dripping. Place the sausages in the batter and put the tin into a hot oven (200°C, 400°F, Gas 6) for approximately 40 minutes.

Irish stew

Serves 2   carbohydrates per portion: 25

225 g (8 oz) best end lamb
225 g (8 oz) potatoes, peeled
1 large onion, peeled and finely sliced
450 ml (¾ pint) stock or water
14 g (½ oz) pearl barley
salt and pepper

Cut up the meat into 2·5-cm (1-in) cubes and remove any excess fat. Chop up the potatoes, if very large. Put the meat, potatoes and onion into a pan, add the water and barley and bring to the boil. Skim well and leave to simmer for 1½ hours on top of the stove. Check seasoning and serve piping hot.

Tripe and onions

Serves 2   carbohydrates per portion: 20

350 g (¾ lb) tripe   ½ tablespoon cornflour
2 large onions   pinch ground mace
300 ml (½ pint) low-fat milk   salt and pepper

Wash the tripe and cut into 5-cm (2-in) squares. Peel the onions and slice finely. Add three-quarters of the milk to a saucepan, in which you have placed the tripe and onions. Season with mace and bring to the boil. Leave to simmer for 30–45 minutes until the tripe is tender. Add the cornflour to the remaining milk and blend thoroughly. Pour this mixture into the tripe and bring to the boil, simmering until the sauce has thickened. Adjust seasoning and serve.

Whiting en papillotes

Serves 2   carbohydrates per portion: 14

2 medium-sized whiting
1 small onion
25 g (1 oz) butter

1 tablespoon dried herbs
2 tablespoons white wine
salt and pepper

Clean the whiting and remove the guts. Dry thoroughly both the cavity and the outside with kitchen paper. Peel and finely slice the onion. Place a small knob of butter, ½ tablespoon dried herbs and half the onion slices inside the cavity of each fish. Season with salt and pepper. Place each fish in a piece of silver foil, dot with butter and pour over 1 tablespoon of white wine. Wrap up the parcels so that they are airtight. Place in a baking dish and put into a moderate oven (180°C. 350°F, Gas 4) for 30 minutes. Remove from the tin foil and serve immediately.

Courgettes stuffed with shrimps

Serves 4   carbohydrates per portion: 0

4 medium-sized courgettes, weighing roughly
    100 g (4 oz) each
225 g (8 oz) shrimps
2 tablespoons lemon juice
black pepper
slices of lemon for garnish

Put the courgettes into boiling salted water and cook for about 10 minutes. Drain. Dig out a hole in each courgette big enough so that you can fill them with the shrimps, lemon juice and black pepper. Garnish with slices of lemon. This makes a light but satisfying main course for the slimmer.

Puddings

Raspberry fool

Serves 4   carbohydrates per portion: 8

350 g (¾ lb) raspberries
2 tablespoons water
liquid sweetener to taste
2 cartons natural yoghurt (5 fl oz size)

Rinse the raspberries and put them into a saucepan with the water. Cook over a gentle heat for a few minutes until you have a thick pulp. Put this pulp through a sieve to remove the pips. Add liquid sweetener to taste and leave to cool. Then stir in the yoghurt and serve well chilled.

Baked egg custard

Serves 4   carbohydrates per portion: 8

3 large eggs
600 ml (1 pint) milk made from low fat powder
½ teaspoon vanilla esence
6–8 drops liquid sweetener
pinch nutmeg

Break the eggs into an overproof dish and beat lightly with a fork. In a small saucepan, heat the milk and add the vanilla essence. Do not allow to boil. Stir into the egg mixture and sprinkle the top with nutmeg. Place the dish in a tray of water and bake in a cool oven (150°C, 300°F, Gas 2) for about 1 hour. The custard should just be set.

Apple snow

Serves 4   carbohydrates per portion: 10

450 g (1 lb) cooking apples   2 egg whites
juice and zest of 1 lemon   liquid sweetener to taste

Cut a shallow incision round the middle of each apple. Put
them in a baking dish and bake in a moderate oven (180°C,
350°F, Gas 4) for 30 minutes. Remove the pulp from the
apples and put this through a sieve. Add liquid sweetener
to taste. Leave the mixture to cool. Meanwhile, beat the
egg whites until stiff and then add the apple pulp a little at a
time. Put into decorative dishes, leave to chill thoroughly
and serve.

Chocolate mousse

Serves 4   carbohydrates per portion: 8

100 g (4 oz) plain cooking chocolate
25 g (1 oz) softened butter
1 tablespoon brandy
juice of 1 Seville orange
4 egg whites

Break up the chocolate into an ovenproof dish and put in a
warm oven to melt. When melted, stir in the butter,
brandy and orange juice. Then leave to cool whilst beating
the egg whites until stiff. Fold the chocolate mixture into
the egg whites as swiftly as possible and pour into ramekin
dishes. Leave to chill in the fridge and serve.

Lemon soufflé

Serves 4   carbohydrates per portion: 12 -

4 eggs, separated   juice and zest of 1 lemon
3 tablespoons castor sugar

Beat the yolks of the eggs with the sugar and grated lemon
rind and juice for several minutes until light and frothy.
Whip the egg whites until stiff and fold them into the
lemon mixture. Pour into a buttered soufflé dish and bake
in a hot oven (200°C, 400°F, Gas 6) for 10 minutes. The
making of this dish should be done as quickly as possible.

Easy calculations for carbohydrate values

The following is a list which should help you to calculate the values of different foods very quickly; it is done in carbohydrate units, one unit being 10 grammes of available carbohydrate. (Thus, a food listed in the carbohydrate counter section as having a value of 10 grammes of carbohydrate for one ounce, given that one ounce is the portion one would normally eat, will be listed below as having one carbohydrate unit.) The British Diabetic Association of 10 Queen Anne Street, London W1, call these 'exchange units' and counting in these units may help those of you suffering from diabetes. (Professor John Yudkin and other dieticians use 5 grammes of available carbohydrate to the carbohydrate unit.) If working in units of 10 grammes, and your daily allowance is, say, 350 grammes, then according to this list of units, your intake should not exceed 35.

	carbohydrate units per average portion
All-Bran	1·5
Apple, eating	1
Banana, peeled	2
Beefburger, ¼lb or 100g	1
Blancmange	2
Bread, 1 slice, white or brown	1·5
Castle pudding	5
Cheeseburger	2
Chicken and ham pie	3
Chop suey	3
Christmas pudding	2
Cornflakes	1·5
Cottage pie	2
Doughnut	3
Fish cakes	2
Fruit mousse	1
Fruit salad, tinned	2
Gingerbread	2
Grapefruit, half	0·5
Grapenuts	1·5
Haddock, fried in breadcrumbs	2
Haggis	2
Ham, chopped loaf	4
Hamburger, ¼lb or 100g	0·5
Honey, 1 spoonful on toast, etc	1
Lancashire hot-pot	1
Ice-cream, plain vanilla	2
Jam omelette	3
Jelly, fruit	2
Junket	2
Kedgeree	3
Lentil soup	1
Macaroni cheese	25
Melon	1

Mince pies	4
Mutton chop, fried	1
Nectarine	1·5
Oatmeal, porridge	1
Orange	1·5
Paella	3
Peach	1
Pear	1
Pineapple	1
Pizza	6
Plum pudding	5
Puffed Wheat	2
Ravioli	3
Rice Krispies	2·5
Sago pudding	2
Sausages, pork, fried	2
Scampi, fried in batter	12
Scotch egg	1
Shepherd's pie	2
Shredded Wheat	1·5
Shreddies	1·5
Spaghetti Bolognese	2
Suet pudding	5
Sugar Puffs	2·5
Swiss apple pudding	4
Vita-Weat	1
Weetabix	2·5
Yoghurt, fruit-flavoured	2
Yorkshire pudding	1·5